TEN SECRETS

A HEALTHCARE QUALITY IMPROVEMENT HANDBOOK

DAVID KASHMER

SARAH CANNON

MICHELE WOLF

JARVIS GRAY

& WALTER HAYNE

TABLE OF CONTENTS

Foreword

Our nation's healthcare is by far the most expensive in the world. In Washington, a recent aim of reform is not just to extend medical coverage to everybody but also to bring costs under control.

Spending on doctors, hospitals, drugs, and the like now consumes more than one of every six dollars we earn.

Many physicians, including myself, are remarkably oblivious to the financial implications of their decisions. They see their patients. They make their recommendations and send out the bills. And, as long as the numbers come out all right at the end of each month, they put the money out of their minds.

Ten Secrets highlights how, in this era of cost containment and resource allocation, quality of care can be emphasized, enhanced and enriched. It attempts to reconcile the need to generate revenue with the critical need to ensure quality.

Through real life examples from their broad experience, the authors lay out a framework designed to manage complex environments where authority is diffuse. They explain how to lead effectively in a changing healthcare landscape and provide insights that strengthen your abilities to communicate complex ideas on healthcare quality.

Ten Secrets may help to galvanize a dynamic team of people and to create collaborative opportunities. It's a starting point to achieve conflict resolution and management while emphasizing patient care as the ultimate focus.

The authors' combined experiences in the important field of healthcare quality is invaluable and is concisely presented in an easily digestible format with a bullet point summary to conclude each secret.

Just how significant are the costs of poor quality? What is *poka*-yoke? Why is a 99.9% success rate not good enough in healthcare? Are we able to utilize those tools used so effectively in manufacturing and industry in our pursuit of healthcare quality improvement? How do you actually utilize data in a meaningful way to help guide change?

If you are interested in creative, simple and effective solutions that challenge current dogma in this ever-changing landscape of healthcare quality, this book is for you.

Firas G. Madbak, MD, FACS, FCCP

Assistant Professor of Surgery

Division of Acute Care Surgery

Dept. of Surgery

University of Florida-Jacksonville

WHY WE WROTE THIS BOOK

Most service industries create about one defect in every one thousand opportunities at making a defect. Said differently, that means things go off the rails about 1 in every 1000 times a certain thing is performed in a service industry.

Notice how that means 99.9% of the time, things go just fine.

That may *seem* fine in certain industries...like making cheeseburgers or sorting mail. But in high-stakes industries like healthcare, that typical level of defect production isn't ok.

Now we *aren't* saying that industries like cheeseburger-making or sorting mail are unimportant. But we *are* saying that the reduction of that typical defect rate seen in service industries is arguably even more important in healthcare.

After all, if 99.9% were ok in a high-stakes field, we'd have no problem with the idea that there'd be a plane crash just about every day at a busy airport like Logan or Philadelphia International. After all, 99.9% is good enough, right?

In fact, we are saying that 99.9% error-free is *not* ok in healthcare. And in this book, we'll share some key secrets that you can use to help reduce that defect rate no matter what specific tools you're using to try and get the job done.

WHY YOU SHOULD READ THIS BOOK

You may have some idea about just how many techniques to improve healthcare quality exist out there.

Whether it's Lean, Six Sigma, Lean Six Sigma or one of the other host of quality toolboxes out there, you probably have come into contact with a quality improvement system before you ever picked up this book.

With all of the toolsets out there, our team has seen *many* ways that quality improvement projects or other deployments can go very wrong very quickly. Or sometimes just have no impact at all other than to waste a great deal of time, money, and effort.

This work, created by National Malcolm Baldrige Quality Award Examiners, Lean Six Sigma Master Black Belts, and practicing clinicians focuses you squarely on how to avoid important pitfalls that will thwart your quality improvement efforts.

Here are ten secrets to help you avoid failure in your work to improve healthcare quality in your practice, hospital, or healthcare system.

Secret One: You Need A Better Definition of Healthcare Quality Improvement

One of the biggest problems we see with teams that set out to improve healthcare relates to how they *think* about healthcare quality.

Intuitive definitions of healthcare quality, like "I know what quality is when I see it" or "quality is adhering to published guidelines" often fail to capture many of the important things that impact both patients and the bottom line of an individual organization.

In particular, failure to understand a useful definition of healthcare quality often leaves the team wondering who exactly it serves in its healthcare quality improvement efforts.

Does the quality effort serve the patient's interest? Is it the third-party payer's? Whose measuring stick is the one the project needs to satisfy?

Unlike other industries, the stakeholders often don't line up...and sometimes they even conflict. For that reason, it's extraordinarily important to have a rigorous, clear, and applicable definition of what healthcare quality improvement exactly. A good definition, applied correctly, actually can resolve many of the problems that doom healthcare quality projects from the start.

Here's one that's useful: healthcare quality improvement is systematic reduction of the variation in output, sometimes accompanied by adjusting the central tendency of a system, as measured against specification limits from the third-party payer, patient, or other important recipient of the system output—whichever is the most difficult to satisfy.

Now let's unpack that definition together.

First, you need to come to accept the fact that there is a standard approach to quality improvement based on tools that apply for all service industries and all manufacturing industries. These tools are agnostic. They don't know or care which industry they represent.

However, failure to adopt and understand these tools as well as failure to apply them appropriately in healthcare has led to confusion and at times rejection of these as the standard approaches. In fact, sometimes we often see healthcare colleagues reinventing tools that already exist!

So take a moment and accept the idea that, unfortunately, healthcare is probably about a decade behind other industries (at least) when it comes to quality improvement. Now back to the show on the definition.

Healthcare quality improvement is the systematic reduction of the variation in output of a system, sometimes accompanied by adjusting the central tendency of the system, as measured against specification limits from the third-party payer, patient, or other important recipient of the system output—whichever is the most difficult to satisfy.

Every output from every system demonstrates some distribution. There is some dispersion, some range of values, for outputs for that system.

Sometimes, these outputs are normally distributed. That's a special kind of outputs seen sometimes, and you may have learned about it as a "bell curve" or "Gaussian distribution". Sometimes they're not.

For our purposes here, it's really not important. But what *is* important is for you to understand that a wider spread of outcomes seen isn't a good thing. In other words, variation is bad. We want a narrow distribution or range of outputs that we seen.

Reduction in the range of outputs seen means there's an improved quality.

Failure to think of quality this way leads teams to focus on averages, like Average Length of Stay, and *average* time to turn over an OR room.

Focusing exclusively on the average (one measure of central tendency of the date) leads to predictable problems. Although decreasing the average can be very helpful (it's in the definition of healthcare quality improvement that we shared) the fact is that focusing on the average for different healthcare systems leads to some predictable problems.

Although the average is important, it's often not the killer. The killer in a system is the spread of outputs seen. In fact, we see *many* projects which decrease the average length of stay (for example) but, unfortunately, still don't make a big impact because the spread (variation) in length of stay is so great that *many* patients still stay too long...and *those* patients are the ones causing the issue for the hospital.

So one issue is that, because teams often have a bad definition of quality improvement, they focus on averages rather than decreasing variation. And healthcare has some other unique challenges too.

It's important for healthcare teams to understand who sets the specification limits against which they measure these outputs—and *that* can be a very difficult task. Who exactly sets the bar for what is called too long, too slow, or too lousy...and who decides exactly what a defect is?

Sometimes, third-party payers clearly specify a limit on time, space, infection rate, or whatever it is the team is trying to improve. Sometimes their voice is the one that matters.

Sometimes, patients specify the mark that the team is trying to do better than. Sometimes, the government or another controlling entity specifies the output.

The challenge, in healthcare, is that sometimes (actually often) these voices all differ. Well now what?

The definition we shared includes the idea that, in healthcare, we should measure ourselves against whichever stakeholder is the most difficult to satisfy.

Whether it's the Voice Of the Patient (VOP), Voice Of the Payer (also VOP), or Voice Of the Legal system (VOL), whichever one sets the most difficult level to satisfy is the one the healthcare team should try to meet.

After all, we have to satisfy these often conflicting specification limits anyhow. Measuring improvement against the toughest means the others get satisfied too.

So now you know: a better definition of healthcare quality improvement recognizes the multiple stakeholders in addition to the systematic reduction of variation in the system.

SUMMARY

- How teams think about quality improvement often leads to predicable failures.

- Recognizing healthcare quality improvement as the systematic reduction of variation in a system, not just changing a central tendency like the average, makes it more likely your project will succeed.

- Quality improvement tools don't really care what industry they're being used in or system they're being used on, *but in healthcare they need to be applied in a certain way.*

- One of the special issues in healthcare is selecting which stakeholder sets the bar. Is it the patient, the third party payer, the government, the legal system...who is it exactly?!

- Selecting the stakeholder's specification that is the most difficult to satisfy, the "voice" that is the toughest to satisfy, helps improve the chance that your project will succeed.

Secret Two: The Tools You're Using For Quality Improvement Aren't Good Enough. (And Here Are Some Better Ones.)

We often see lousy tools used in healthcare for quality improvement. Sometimes, teams even reinvent ones that already exist because they don't have a deep understanding of what quality improvement means or just lack familiarity with standard techniques.

Like we shared in the first chapter, often teams don't recognize reducing variation as a hallmark (perhaps *the* hallmark) of quality improvement.

Maybe owing to that, healthcare quality teams often rely on tools that also failed to recognize this fact.

Again, there's that classic focus on average length of stay. Teams talk about average time to the operating room... However, these tools just don't cut it for all the reasons talked about previously in Secret One.

When teams do use some standard tools, they often don't apply them correctly.

For example, you may have heard of a control chart. It makes perfect sense when you read about a control chart that you may want to use this on your process as part of your improvement project.

After all, a control chart may tell you whether you have a process that is in statistical control or out of control. We'll leave it at that for now.

Here's the problem: if you apply a control chart to a system that is making defects, the control chart may show you that the system is in control.

In other words, there is no unexpected or changing variation in your system. However, ut-oh, your system may continue to produce an unacceptable output...even though the control chart demonstrates that the system is "in control".

And that's the problem: the control chart may make you think everything is *fine.* It really is just telling you that your process will continue to produce that same output predictably and routinely...but it will not tell you whether that output is acceptable.

It also won't tell you a measure for how incapable your process is when it comes to performing adequately.

That particular foul with control charts, where it misleads a team into thinking all is well because things are "in control", is one that we see all the time.

The issue? A lack of understanding of classic quality improvement tools.

Whether we are using tools that fail to recognize variation, or whether we use tools sporadically and inappropriately, this secret to is all about the fact that healthcare is often way off the mark when it comes to using standard quality tools.

So then what are some classic, useful tools for healthcare?

CPK's, Sigma values, tests that demonstrate significant decreases in variation from a process. There are *many*.

The specifics on each of these is beyond the scope of this book. But those are just a few. Using them, and using them correctly in healthcare, takes training, expertise, and time.

We mention them here so that you know they're out there, and so that you remember the tests don't care whether they are applied to a process in healthcare or some other industry. Just so long as they're used properly.

It's about time we learn them and use them routinely.

SUMMARY

- Failure to know, understand, and apply standard quality improvement tools leads to all sorts of problems in healthcare quality projects...including the occasional reinvention of tools that already exist!

- When teams *do* attempt to use standard tools, they often focus on things like averages and mis-apply tools owing to lack of familiarity, expertise, or both.

- A classic example is the application of a control chart to a process *prior* to working to improve a process.

The control chart may say that the process is performing in its routine fashion…even if that routine fashion includes the reliable production of defects!

- Specific tools include creating CPK values, sigma values, KW tests, ANOVA, and *many* others. Although the specifics are outside the scope of this book, the bottom line is that these tools are out there and expertise can help teams apply them properly.

SECRET THREE: LOTS OF PLACES LOVE LEAN, BUT LEAN ALONE ISN'T GOOD ENOUGH...

When we say "lots of places love Lean", we mean llloooovvvveeee Lean.

And the truth is, Lean is great. It works on decreasing the eight wastes seen in organizations.

Those can be remembered with the acronym DOWNTIME: Defects, Overproduction, Waiting, Non-utilized talent, Time, Inventory, Motion, and Extra processing.

Here's the thing though: it seems like healthcare loves Lean because there is so much waste that just about any template for quality improvement will work. Let us explain...

Healthcare is sooo far behind when in comes to quality improvement that even the more basic quality tools (many of which are included in Lean) will achieve a good effect. There's *lots* of low-hanging fruit.

And so Lean can help us get past the lower levels of quality improvement.

However, the Lean by itself only gets us so far. To say otherwise doesn't match our experience and the knowledge base from additional quality improvement training.

Let's be clear before all the zealots who believe in Lean only (to the exclusion of all else) go on the attack: Lean is *very* useful in healthcare.

That's especially true because healthcare as an industry is in its infancy (or at best early adolescence) in terms of quality improvement.

However, Lean tools alone and are nowhere near enough for advanced quality improvement. Want to get at the higher levels of quality? Wondering *why* you haven't seen everything you expected from a Lean deployment? Often, that's because Lean isn't enough all by itself.

Sure, Lean may be less "mathy" or "math-intense" than other quality systems...but daily huddles and pretty drawings only get you so far. Remember: Lean has some nice, basic tools...which can really help you when you first begin to really focus on quality.

Truth is, Lean needs to be coupled with other advanced tools so the variation can be seen and understood.

How do we know? Because we've done it. We've lived with Lean and we've seen it deployed to varying effects when it's set out all by itself.

And the variations on Lean that we typically see deployed in healthcare are great for bringing people together, forming teams, surfacing issues, and to promote flow...

But to get at higher levels of quality improvement, we need the additional tools beyond just the very useful ones of Lean.

Again, the secret here: Lean can really help healthcare quality improvement... because healthcare quality improvement has so far to go.

If we really want to get to the next level of excellence, we need tools beyond just Lean.

SUMMARY

- Some health systems love Lean...sometimes even to the exclusion of all else.

- Healthcare as a field is early in its quality improvement journey.

- Lean is a useful toolset, but part of the reason why is because healthcare has such a long way to go in terms of quality improvement.

- Lean works, in part, by targeting the 8 wastes, which can be remembered as DOWNTIME.

- Lean tools alone don't work as well for visualizing defect and variation in a system. Sometimes this leaves a team wondering why defects are still being made so frequently despite Lean improvements.

- Lean tools alone are not enough to move beyond the low-hanging fruit of healthcare quality improvement.

SECRET FOUR: WE NEED BETTER ACCOUNTING TOOLS TO SHOW THE TRUE COSTS OF POOR QUALITY

In business school, you learn a lot about accounting.

...and in medical school, as well as other health professional schools, you learn pretty much nothing about accounting.

However, in both cases, you learn very little about how accounting works when it comes to costs that result from poor quality.

In fact, typical accounting courses don't teach you anything about how poor quality can be captured from some of the classic financial statements that an organization is using.

This shortcoming makes it a very difficult in healthcare to capture the costs associated with poor quality (COPQ).

It's consistently amazing to our team that healthcare institutions don't realize just how much is walking out the door owing to poor quality.

In fact, failure to adequately represent costs lost to poor quality means it's very hard to do things like justify spending money on quality. It's even harder to be assured that, if we do spend money on quality, will see a return on that investment.

For that reason, it's important to understand two things. First, cost can be used as a measure of waste. It's especially useful because people in the C suite, physicians, and many different stakeholders in the hospital can understand what it means when we talk about the waste measure called cost.

Costs, particularly the Costs of Poor Quality (COPQ), is a measure of waste that can be understood by physicians, other caregivers, the C-suite, and multiple stakeholders across a healthcare organization.

For physicians, there are obviously other measures of waste they sometimes find more intuitive.

These may include extra days in the hospital, nosocomial infections, and multiple other things that really hurt patients.

However, it's very useful to think of waste in terms of cost as this spans stakeholders.

With a little education, physicians, the C suite, and many other hospital groups can understand and get their heads around costs (specifically the COPQ) as a measure of waste.

The second thing it's important to understand is that there are defined ways in which the costs lost to poor quality can be teased out from balance sheets and, more typically, income statements.

The profit and loss statement can be utilized to construct what's called that cost of poor quality. It's something our team has written about previously, and it's worth having a look:

http://bit.ly/COPQWriteUp

One way to think of it is that the cost of poor quality (again, COPQ) is composed of four buckets.

These include internal failures, external failures, cost of surveillance, and costs of prevention.

Importantly each of those four buckets has a clear definition.

The cost of internal failures includes all of the failures that happen in the system but don't actually make it to the patient.

Or, if you're focusing a quality project on another stakeholder (like billing the third party payer) you can think of internal failures portion of the COPQ as the costs associated when a defect happens but doesn't make it to the third party payer, *eg* a claim that isn't made properly and has to be re-worked before going out the door.

Similarly, by the way, if your project is focused on a stakeholder other than the patient, you'll need to adjust all the buckets that we're about to describe to be centered around the stakeholder you're doing the project for.

In our description, we'll keep on using the COPQ as it relates to patients, because that's how we use it most commonly.

Examples of internal failures typically include wasted medications, extra motion, extra inventory, time used in reworking something, and numerous other failings.

In contrast, the cost of external failures is often much more visible and memorable. The costs in this bucket tend to be the ones focused on in many quality improvement groups.

These are dramatic and represent what happens when a defect makes it to the patient. This may be, for example, costs associated with mis-dosing a medication.

It may be dosing a patient on a medication to which they are allergic only to have the patient's condition greatly worsen.

Again, external failures are typically more dramatic, in general, than the other buckets. They may garner a great deal of attention.

External failures are sometimes useful as the impetus to start a quality improvement project.

It's always interesting, incidentally, that focusing on the non-spectacular internal failures often gets us much further than concentrating on the external ones.

After all, making it so that no defects make it to the patient by reducing internal failures often eliminates the need to drill down on external failures.

Even though that seems to be the case, staff aren't as engaged by unspectacular work like eliminating drawing up the wrong medication and not dosing it to the patient. That kind of work is non-glamorous. But, truth is, doing just that is how quality gets improved!

Whatever the case, internal failures and external failures are not the only two important buckets. There are two others.

Another important bucket is the cost of surveillance. The cost of surveillance includes all those costs associated with checking up on a system owing to the fact that it produces defects.

This may include time spent by nursing in order to review paperwork time and time again with the knowledge that the paperwork is typically defective.

It may include an accrediting body like the American College of surgeons the needs to return to the trauma center more often to check up on it owing to poor performance.

The cost of surveillance includes, again, all those costs associated with checking up on a system owing to its poor level of performance.

This last bucket category is our favorite. That one is the cost of prevention. This is the only one of the four buckets the returns a positive return on investment when we allocate money to it. It's also one of the least commonly utilized buckets.

The only COPQ bucket with a positive return on investment is the prevention bucket. Spending resources on prevention may have (and often does have) a positive return on investment.

We rarely see money intentionally spent in healthcare on preventing defects.

Even moreso, we rarely see money spent to prevent defects with a strong intention that there will be a return.

However, the cost of prevention include those costs associated with heading defects off at the pass.

Examples here may include the cost of a new medication review system that helps decrease the chance that a patient with an allergy will be dosed on that medication.

However, it's especially important that the finance team be involved with any group looking to improve quality so that the two groups can get together on what the actual costs of poor quality are. This makes for a better estimate of what any project can recover.

In the end, the point of this secret is that in healthcare we often measure waste with multiple yardsticks if we measure it at all.

That's why the cost of poor quality is a great, easily understandable measure. It cuts across the C suite and other stakeholders so that we can get a better sense of exactly how much waste is occurring in the system that we're looking at.

Here's a hint: when we use the cost of poor quality, we typically find that any proposed healthcare quality improvement project returns approximately $320,000-$350,000 per year. It's *amazing* just how much waste there is.

And when we hold this up next to potential Medicare withholds, we realize that several good quality improvement projects return an amount that is often on par with what we stand to lose from Medicare and other third-party payer clawbacks.

And, of course, improving quality not only recovers that amount...it also leads to improvement in the very endpoints that Medicare uses to claw back reimbursement. That's why quality projects and using the COPQ is far superior to simply focusing on the typically more visible amount you stand to lose to Medicare on different endpoints.

SUMMARY

- It can be very difficult to capture the waste associated with poor quality in healthcare owing to lack of education or the presence of multiple stakeholders with different interests.

- The COPQ (Cost of Poor Quality) is a standard approach that lets multiple different hospital groups understand the waste present in the system.

- The COPQ is composed of four buckets, including the costs of:

    o Internal failures (problems that DON'T make it to the patient or stakeholder that you're focusing on)

    o External failures (defects that DO make it to the patient or stakeholder)

    o Surveillance (costs of having to check up on a lousy system)

    o Prevention (costs incurred when spending money to prevent problems in the first place)

- When it comes to poor quality, the internal failures are often MUCH less dramatic than the external failures. Use external failures as rallying cries when you decide to start a project, because staff understand what it means when a patient has something bad happened to them.

28

- Even though internal failures are not spectacular, eliminating those helps eliminate external failures. They're not glamorous but they are often the way ahead in quality improvement in healthcare.

- A typical COPQ for almost any project in healthcare (even one at smaller centers) is $300,000 to $350,000. It's amazing how things add up quickly in healthcare.

- Although potential withholding from Medicare gets a lot of attention, just a few good quality projects often recover just as much as we could potentially lose from Medicare clawbacks AND of course the project itself often improves Medicare endpoints if aligned properly.

Secret Five: Don't Choose a Bad Solution

With every quality project, we typically get the chance to choose solutions or interventions to help improve our system.

And this is another place where teams typically fall down.

How? They choose a lousy solution.

Knowing what bad solutions look like can help protect you against their siren call. If you know what to look out for, you hopefully won't be lulled into choosing an intervention that's doomed to fail.

Before we get to specifics, let's talk for a minute about a useful concept called *poka-yoke.*

Some translations of the Japanese term are something like "idiot proofing".

A better way to think of that design philosophy is as making it easier to do the right thing and difficult, if not impossible, to do the wrong thing.

Poka-yoke is the idea that our quality interventions should make it easier to do the right thing and impossible to do the wrong thing.

That design philosophy is *much* different than what we typically see in healthcare quality improvement projects.

What do we often see?

Another checksheet. Or another piece of paper. Or a memory intensive multi-step process to notify many people about something.

And the solutions often rely on the provider (doctor, nurse, advanced practitioner) to execute the plan.

Sure, they may be in the middle of an emergency, or swamped with the 60% of their day that already includes pushing paper, and yet quality teams often feel adding one more piece of paper to the provider's busy day will somehow improve things.

Guess what. It often doesn't.

It's just a lazy approach to creating a solution. We can come up with better solutions in healthcare.

Poka-yoke as an approach to choosing solutions helps us think much differently.

For example: are people not present for the time-out in your OR? What about using a rule that the patient can not be moved to the OR table until all team members are present?

Do people skip portions of the OR checklist? What about a visual control that keeps the team focused on all parts?

Regardless of solutions that you think may work in your organization, you can see that bad solutions have certain characteristics.

Where *poka-yoke* makes us think about solutions like "hmmm, if we keep running out of wheelchairs what if we made it so that wheelchairs just couldn't fit out the door?" typical thinking in healthcare is more like "we should have a 10 item paper for the charge nurse to complete prior to wheelchair request and then the nurse should call central supply..."

Yuck—that second one is a bad solution!

So now you know: a good solution is one which is easy to execute, happens often automatically, and does NOT add to administrative burden. In fact sometimes a good solution could *lessen* paperwork—when was the last time you saw *that* happen in healthcare?

There are some other characteristics too: the solution should be durable, meaning it keeps working long-term even when you aren't looking at it. (Is creating a new paper and multiple phone calls durable or just a recipe for burn-out?)

Another important characteristic is that the solution should be measurable in an easy fashion. Meaning there should be some way to tell whether it's being used or doing what it's supposed to do, and it should be easy to check in on it.

One last characteristic for a good solution that is *very* important in healthcare: the solution should work on nights, weekends, holidays...all those times when sick patients come to the hospital and resources are even more scarce.

Don't imagine your solution working at noon on a weekday when you have a cup of coffee in your hand and full staff around you.

Imagine it working on Christmas Eve at midnight in a snowstorm.

What we've described are just several characteristics of a good solution, and they all fit with that *poka-yoke* design philosophy.

Adjust things so that it's easier to do the right thing, difficult (if not impossible) to do the wrong thing, and to keep on doing the right thing over and over again.

Summary

- Knowing what bad solutions look like can help us choose better interventions to improve quality.

- *Poka-yoke* is the design philosophy that helps guide staff to choose solutions that make it easier to do the right thing and difficult, if not impossible, to make a defect.

- Bad solutions include ones that increase paperwork, rely completely on busy practitioners, don't work in early AM hours or weekends, and are difficult to check in on to make sure they are still working.

- Imagine how your potential solution would work at 3AM on Christmas day when it's snowing—not on a sunny weekday when the hospital is fully staffed, it's sunny outside, and you're holding a cup of fresh coffee.

- Select an intervention that will keep on working over time. It's worthwhile to find a durable solution.

SECRET SIX: A JOB DONE 99.9% CORRECT IS NOT GOOD ENOUGH IN HEALTHCARE

Like we discussed earlier, most service industries operate at a 99.9% error-free rate.

Said differently, there's only about one defect made per every thousand opportunities at making a defect in most service industries.

Intuitively, that seems great and feels very good on a day-to-day basis. Only rarely do things seem to go wrong.

Again, intuitively, 99.9% may feel "good enough".

However, unfortunately, for high-stakes industries like healthcare 99.9% just isn't ok. If that defect rate were good enough, then

- Two short or long landings at most major airports each day

- 200,000 wrong prescriptions each year

- no electricity for about 7 hours per month

would all be perfectly acceptable.

Basically, in things that matter, 99.9% correct just isn't good enough. And healthcare is something that matters.

And now you know: typical process performance, even if it feels like things are great, is totally unacceptable in high-stakes fields like healthcare and aviation.

SUMMARY

- Processes in service industries typically operate at 1 defect per one thousand opportunities at making a defect.

- While that rate may *feel* fine, it turns out that rate is not acceptable for high stakes fields like healthcare.

- Don't think that, just because a healthcare system "feels" fine, that performance is just fine.

SECRET SEVEN: LOTS OF PEOPLE IN HEALTHCARE HAVE OPINIONS ON QUALITY, & FEW HAVE EDUCATION ON IT

This secret is going to be a tough one for some readers. We think of it as the "tough love" section of the book.

And this secret just is what it is: lots of people in healthcare including practitioners, administrators, and many others want to comment all about quality—but have no education in quality as a field.

True, there are many different types of education regarding how to improve quality. However, it's consistently impressive how many people who hold positions in quality improvement lack substantive education on exactly the basics of quality and what quality means.

We routinely seen people who run entire quality departments who have not only *no* experience in quality improvement but who lack even the roots of education regarding quality.

Sometimes these are excellent practitioners, intelligent colleagues, or highly experienced individuals...often all three. But experienced and educated in quality improvement? Often the answer is no.

This seems to be fairly prevalent in healthcare. That may be because healthcare requires such a substantial amount of education to enter the field at all that any more education is viewed as particularly difficult to obtain in terms of time and money.

For whatever reason, many in healthcare feel like they know what quality is when they see it, or try to achieve quality on a case by case basis rather than looking to decrease variation in a system. (See Secret 1.)

Regardless of the exact reasons, it just seems to be the many in healthcare lack education in the basics of quality improvement, and this leads to many different issues.

For example, there is often no common language about quality because staff are unable to assume a common ground owing to the fact that the language and tools of quality remain unknown or unused.

Other difficulties include the fact that healthcare often reinvents the wheel.

Unfortunately, healthcare often tries to re-invent the wheel when it comes to the use of quality tools. When it does, it generally creates versions of the tools that are very inferior to the original tried-and-true tools. And that's often because of a lack of knowledge about the tools that are out there.

By this we mean that some basic quality tools that easily apply to healthcare simply are not used because healthcare as a field is largely unaware of them. The field then goes on to create tools very similar (yet often inferior) to ones that already exist and work.

Often these new tools are one-offs seen in a journal entry or something similar.

Our feeling is we're likely able to do better as a field by using standard quality tools and implementing them properly in healthcare.

Again, the tools don't know which field they're in. What we mean by that is it's not as if the tools just work in manufacturing or just work in other service industries but can't/don't work in healthcare.

That's simply not correct and reflects a fundamental misunderstanding of the nature of many of the tools used by quality improvement. Why is that?

Again, likely because there is little to no education on the basics of quality in healthcare.

As a result, quality tools and systems are often viewed with skepticism. Quality improvement tools are often viewed as not easily applicable to healthcare or only applicable to manufacturing.

Again these issues may have their roots in a fundamental lack of understanding of exactly what quality is born from a lack of education and quality improvement tools.

The solution? Education, practice, and patience.

Remember, one of the toughest things everyone faces is to have a sense of what they don't know.

If you're at all unsure whether this secret describes you, no problem! Get in touch with a quality professional and let them help.

SUMMARY

- This is the tough love section of the book.

- Lots of people in healthcare have opinions on quality & very few have education in the field. Don't be one of those people.

- This leads to lack of a common language about quality in the field of healthcare.

- This also leads to reinventing the wheel, where healthcare teams re-create known quality tools (often inferior versions of known tools) or fail to use standard tools at all. This leads to missed opportunities or inappropriate conclusions.

- The idea that standard quality tools can't work in healthcare, expressed as "Lean is great for manufacturing but can't work in healthcare" or something similar, demonstrates this lack of education in quality improvement tools.

- Quality tools don't know or care what field they are used in. Whether a manufacturing field or a service field, the tools are agnostic and the math is the math.

- If you're not sure at all whether this secret describes you, get some education from a professional.

SECRET EIGHT: DATA FROM A DATABASE ISN'T AS USEFUL FOR QUALITY IMPROVEMENT

You may think: "Really? But we have *sooo* much data in healthcare! And now you're saying it's not as useful for healthcare quality improvement?"

Yes, that's exactly what we are saying. And here's why.

First, when you decide on a project, one of the typical steps you take is to define clearly and exactly what endpoints you're going to use. And what each one means specifically. At least, if you want to be successful you do.

So, creating or selecting that operational definition for each endpoint the team will use is very important.

The trouble with data from a database? One important problem is that the operational definition of what you really need to measure often does not align with what's in the database.

One important problem is that the operational definition of what you really need to measure often does not align with what's in the database.

One classic example: Emergency Department (ED) throughput.

Once upon a time, a hospital *really* wanted to improve how long patients waited in the ED after the decision had been made to admit. After all, being in the ED was difficult for both patients and providers. Busy staff would often have to take care of patients who were more acutely ill or for whom there was no diagnosis yet.

The patients who were to be admitted were typically diagnosed and treatment had started.

The result? Patients in the ED who were admitted to the hospital didn't always get their antibiotics, labs, and additional treatments in a timely fashion.

The hospital decided the best move was to decrease how long patients waited in the ED.

And so they started a project. And the hospital administration measured ED throughput for months and months. They created all sorts of policies and paperwork and pushed on the providers to "get those patients admitted faster."

Five months later the ED throughput numbers looked better…but the same problems kept happening. Septic patients didn't seem to be getting those antibiotics any faster. And, although every saw that throughput *looked* better, well, hmmm...things didn't feel any different in the ER when it came to patients waiting to go upstairs to the rest of the hospital.

The only thing that felt different is that people were more tense, angry, and focused on throughput.

What happened?

What had happened was bad data from the database, and here's how.

The database measured time in the ED alright. And it did that by subtracting the time of patient arrival from the time that the order to admit the patient went into the computer.

See the problem? The time in the ED had nothing to do with the actual time that the patient took up space in the ED.

If that example sounds familiar to you, don't worry: this same problem repeats all across many hospitals in the United States.

And this is one reason why database data *seems* so attractive: it's there, we have it, and it's pretty easy to get the electronic health record to spit it out.

Unfortunately, it's often junk because it's not *really* what we want to know!

The solution: sampling prospectively from the system.

We *know* how to obtain data from a system via sampling. We *know* how to select a sample of patients that represent the system overall—it's one of the basic parts of many quality improvement plans.

If we choose a sample that actually represents the system, and obtain data prospectively, guess what: we are often *much* better off.

How do we choose a sample that represents the system? Well, when it comes to EDs for example, we include the tough times and not just the ones that are easy.

By this we mean that the sample includes nights and weekends. Warm sunny days and rainy ones too. The sample we choose has to *actually* represent the ED...not just the good times when we stroll through the ED at noon with coffee in hand.

Specifics of sampling, including selecting sample size, require some quality education and often a quality professional. Not sure how to do it? We share some resources (and our team's email for questions) at the end of the book.

So, the first problem with data from a database is it often does not represent what you *actually* want to know, and so the decisions you make based on the data are of the exact same quality as the data themselves: junk.

But that's not the only problem with data from a database.

Another problem with data from a database is that it's cleaned.

By "cleaned" we mean that extreme values, values make the system look bad, or values that look plain ol' strange are sometimes thrown out before they are recorded in the database.

Another problem with data from a database is that those data are cleaned.

For example, someone in data entry along the way sees that there's a record that a patient was in the ED for three whole days, and the data entry person thinks "that *can't* be right". So that person just leave that value out.

It's not that anyone is trying to cover anything up. It's just that there's a known phenomenon where data that passes through multiple layers before it gets into a database may be cleaned up or otherwise lose fidelity—and therefore its ability to represent your system.

So, is data from a database or warehouse better than nothing? Yes, but only sometimes.

A better option is to prospectively sample what you really need to know and record the values you *actually* get.

Summary

- There's a lot of data collected in healthcare, but unfortunately the data that make it into one of the many databases isn't so great for specifically what you want to look at to improve quality.

- One reason why data from a database isn't great for your healthcare quality improvement project is the fact that the operational definition of the data is different than what you need. It may be called "Time in ED" but it may not be the time the patient is actually in the ED!

- Another reason data from a database isn't so great for your healthcare quality project is that the data are cleaned.

- Sampling prospectively from your system is much more valuable than data from a database. But be sure to obtain a sample that actually represents your system. That means you often need to include nights and weekends in your data collection or you will be misled.

- Is data from a database better than nothing? Yes, but only sometimes. Be careful if you use data from a database so that you aren't misled and so that you don't select an improvement for your system that just won't work.

SECRET NINE: WHEN YOU FEEL YOU DON'T HAVE TIME OR RESOURCES TO COLLECT DATA YOU ARE PROBABLY EVEN MORE IN NEED OF COLLECTING DATA.

It turns out that the systems that are in dire need of data collection also feel like they don't have time or resources to collect data at all.

This is a lesson we've learned from more than one hundred quality improvement projects across more than ten organizations.

Why's that the case? It seems to be that dysfunction after dysfunction, and waste after waste, have piled on top of each other in those systems so much so that the people who work in them can't possibly imagine doing one more thing.

They're busy, or believe they're busy. Unfortunately, despite good intentions (no one wakes up in the morning in healthcare to go to work and do a bad job) the staff are busy in a system that produces defects that often go unnoticed.

So waste abounds and defects continue unnoticed. And wasted time, for one, makes everyone so busy that no one can collect data and meaningfully repair the system.

Or the amount of waste in the system, and continued poor quality, makes it impossible for the system to grow and acquire resources.

Organizations where staff feel they don't have time or resources to collect data (or that it wouldn't matter if they did collect data) are often in the most need of data collection and use.

Unfortunately, without data (and the ability to respond to data) the system continues to be "so busy" that no one could even *think* of collecting data. And in reality it's busy wasting its resources and creating defects.

That's the trouble: the organization can't see its real issues without data, and organizations where the staff feel they are too busy to collect data or that it wouldn't matter if they did anyway are often in the most need.

And the cycle is self-reinforcing: the situation is sometimes dire, and so no one will collect meaningful data on its performance, and so the situation remains dire.

Whether it's understaffing, poor patient care, both, or a host of other issues...it seems that centers which are the most resistant to data collection and use are also in the most need. (See Secret Ten for more reasons why.)

Summary

- In some systems, staff are so knee-deep in waste that they can't imagine collecting data on their processes.

- Unfortunately, failure to collect data leads to the continued unnoticed waste and quality issues.

- This cycle is self-reinforcing: the organization may feel that no one can collect data, and so it remains busy in creating waste, and so believes no one has time to collect data...

- Think you're too busy to collect data? Try not collecting data to make improvements and see how that goes.

Secret Ten: The Ability to Collect, Interpret, and Respond In a Sustained Fashion to Data Is the Mark of an Organization That Is High-functioning

Things *change* in healthcare. Whether that's consolidation of different healthcare systems owing to perceived reimbursed decreases, new initiatives from the government (we're looking at *you* CMS bundled payments), or some other yet-to-be-realized initiative...one thing is for sure: change is the only constant in healthcare.

The trouble is, *many* systems can't respond to changes. We know, because we've worked in those systems.

Whether there are dysfunctional referral systems, inability to provide care for critically ill patients, or an inability to perceive the costs associated with poor quality, the fact is that some healthcare systems are not able to respond when the ground shifts under them and the world looks different.

Sometimes, this is owing to culture. Amazingly, organizational culture is sometimes not aligned with quality initiatives.

In fact, sometimes organizational culture is so maladapted to where things need to go that quality initiatives, data, and data-driven intervention are viewed with skepticism if not outright subversion.

How do we know? We've worked in them. Sometimes they include misaligned physician groups; sometimes they are leadership that doesn't understand what the front lines need...but whichever one of the *many* reasons that culture squelches (or doesn't allow for) substantial quality initiatives, one thing seems constant:

Organizations that can obtain meaningful data, interpret those data, and make sustainable changes to their system (along with performing followup and maintenance on their system) get much further than ones that can't.

Why? Maybe it's because over time more is required of us in healthcare whether by regulation, public sentiment, or both. Whatever the reason, things aren't getting any easier. And changes keep coming quickly.

When we've worked with systems that fall down on any one of the portions of this secret (sometimes it's the inability to collect data, or interpret data, or some other part) it seems like they're eventually washed away.

So this secret is one we share with you to help you preserve and advance your system: look to improve things with data, no matter how good you think you are.

...and if you can't (or don't) understand that fact with time you may be washed away in a wave of regulation.

Summary

- Things change in healthcare. New specifications and requirements are rolled out *all* the time.

- Organizations that lack the ability to obtain data, interpret data, or make sustainable changes to their system based on data will be washed away. Things in healthcare are too complex to think that everything will work out without a rigorous process to understand, adapt, and improve.

- This secret, like many in this book, is based on our experience. And here, the lesson is: without meaningful data, along with the ability to interpret it and make sustainable changes, your healthcare system just has an opinion. And by the time you realize your opinion is incorrect it may be too late. Avoid opinion and learn to use data meaningfully if you can't yet.

- If your culture doesn't align with the use of meaningful data, that culture may not be around much longer.

FAREWELL

With those ten secrets in hand, you've improved your chances for success in your next healthcare quality improvement project.

Whether you help the team understand what quality means, use data directly from the process, or choose solutions that don't add to paperwork or administrative overhead, you're well on your way to getting things done in healthcare quality improvement.

Remember: like many things in life, achieving successful improvement projects is a batting average—many projects won't be home runs, but even a base hit or a walk can really help patients.

So here's to you as you set out to achieve those base hits— the patient's are worth it!

Good luck, and if you have questions say hello to our author team anytime:

info@thehealthcarelab.org

About The Authors

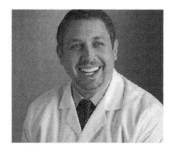 **DAVID KASHMER** is a quality improvement expert, & trauma and acute-care surgeon.

He earned his Medical Doctorate degree from MCP Hahnemann University--now Drexel University College of Medicine--and his Bachelor of Science degree in Biology from Villanova University through a joint BS-MD program with MCP Hahnemann.

He has previously served as a Section Chief, Chief of Surgery, & Chief Medical Officer for healthcare organizations.

David also earned a Lean Six Sigma Master Black Belt certificate at Villanova. Dr. Kashmer holds a Master of Business Administration degree in Healthcare Administration from George Washington University. He recently served on the Board of Examiners for the Malcolm Baldrige National Quality Award.

David has authored multiple books on healthcare quality improvement including several Amazon Bestsellers.

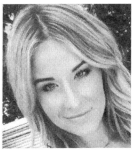

SARAH CANNON focuses on healthcare system organization and helping individuals achieve healthy behaviors. Sarah currently attends the University of North Florida, where her concentration is in Healthcare Administration.

With this and her additional work on improving patient experience, she advocates for high quality healthcare to assist patients in achieving their best possible outcomes.

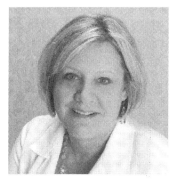

MICHELE WOLF -- Dr. Michele L. Wolf completed her DNP in May 2018 from Maryville University.

Currently, she is an Assistant Professor and the Director of the MSN Program at the University of Tampa.

She also earned a Master of Science in Nursing from the University of Tampa and is nationally certified as a Family Nurse Practitioner.

For the last 10 years, she has practiced as a Family Nurse Practitioner in the Tampa Bay area. She is also a member of Sigma Theta Tau National Honor Society.

Michele's experience in healthcare quality improvement spans more than two decades. Her twenty-year background in Emergency / Trauma nursing helped grow her interest in providing high-quality healthcare.

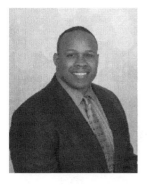 **JARVIS GRAY** is the Chief Improvement Officer and Sr. Managing Director of The Quality Coaching Co.

He offers more than 12 years of quality improvement and project leadership experience in the healthcare industry.

Jarvis has an extensive background in planning and managing cross-functional business operations as well as technology projects.

He earned his Bachelors of Science in Industrial Engineering (BSIE). He additional holds a Master of Healthcare Administration (MHA) degree as well as a Master of Project Management (MPM) degree.

Jarvis is a certified Project Management Professional (PMP) and Manager of Quality & Organizational Excellence (CMQ-OE) through the American Society of Quality (ASQ).

He is also a certified Lean Six Sigma Black Belt (LSSBB) and Malcolm Baldrige National Quality Award Examiner.

Jarvis has managed a broad array of projects across a variety of healthcare settings ranging from inpatient to primary care settings and more.

Prior to launching The Quality Coaching Co., Jarvis held management and senior leader positions centered exclusively on quality and process improvement leadership, project management, and strategic plan execution.

Over the past decade, Jarvis has coached 40+ management and executive leaders in quality and process improvement fundamentals. He has amassed over 2,500 hours of course lecture, training, networking events and public workshops that promote foundations of achieving organizational excellence.

Contact Jarvis at <u>Jarvis.Gray@qualitycoach.org</u>.

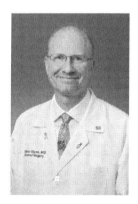

WALTER HAYNE is an experienced General Surgeon and previous Chief of Surgery. He attended college at Temple University after receiving an academic scholarship and went on to receive a scholarship to Temple Medical School in Philadelphia. He completed his residency in General Surgery at Cornell Medical Center's New York Hospital.

Dr. Hayne believes strongly in passing along the knowledge and wisdom of his great mentors. He is currently focused on helping to design and implement a new general surgery residency program.

In addition to training residents, his interests include finding quality improvement solutions that work for practitioners in today's highly regulated, busy medical climate.

His experience with quality improvement in healthcare spans more than two decades.

Dr. Hayne looks to improve quality via adopting best practices and selecting improvements that can be performed by busy practitioners in the field.

OTHER BOOKS FROM THE HEALTHCARE LAB, INC.

<u>Games for Health: Ultimate Beginner's Guide To Using Game Dynamics In Healthcare Organizations</u>

Let's make working in healthcare even more fun...and effective!
There's an engagement crisis among healthcare workers...

According to recent reports, 70% of workers are either not engaged in their work or are actively trying to hurt their company. This lack of engagement leads to missed opportunities, revenue problems, and quality issues. One useful solution is the application of game dynamics to your current system and culture--and this work provides the tools to do just that. Use *Games for Health* to apply game dynamics to healthcare settings in order to facilitate culture change, quality improvement, and better patient care!

<u>Trauma Program Operator's Manual</u>

The Practical, Insider's Guide To Running A Trauma Program

THE TRAUMA PROGRAM OPERATOR'S MANUAL GIVES YOU TOOLS TO SUCCEED!

If you're involved with a trauma program in any way, this manual is for you. It's filled with useful, hard to find info that helps guide your trauma program to excellence and beyond!

Healthcare Information System Hacking: Protect Your System

Understand how your health information is at risk and how hackers attempt to obtain it.

HEALTHCARE INFORMATION SYSTEM HACKING TELLS YOU SPECIFICS ABOUT WHAT YOU NEED TO PROTECT YOUR PRIVATE HEALTH INFORMATION, WHETHER YOU'RE A SYSTEM ADMINISTRATOR, PATIENT, OR HEALTHCARE PROVIDER.

Learn the true value of your health information, and how hackers attempt to access it. *Healthcare Information System Hacking* introduces the specific steps hackers follow to obtain information from a hospital or health system. This book is great for information professionals in healthcare and concerned patients alike!

ONE LAST THING...

If this book was useful to you or if you enjoyed it, we'd really appreciate your review on Amazon.

The support is very important and we do read each and every review so that this work can be updated and improved.

If you're reading the paperback version of the book, we'd appreciate your comments on Amazon.com.

If you're reading this on Kindle, Amazon will ask you for a review. (In just a moment.)

If you enjoyed the book, please take a moment and pass along your feedback!

Made in the USA
Columbia, SC
03 December 2018